HOW TO GROW YOUR HAIR FOR YOUNG AND OLD

15 SIMPLE DIY WAYS TO GROW YOUR HAIR

Amanda R. Branson

TABLE OF CONTENTS

CHAPTER 1

INTRODUCTION

Our hair considerably influences our confidence and self-esteem and plays a vital role in how we look. Hair that is thick and healthy is often equated with youth and attractiveness. Hair loss, on the other hand, is a widespread issue that affects both men and women of all ages. Maintaining optimum hair health requires an understanding of the elements that contribute to healthy hair and the reasons for hair loss.

There are a number of things to take into account when it comes to healthy hair. For the hair follicles to be nourished and to develop, proper nutrition, including a balanced diet rich in vitamins, minerals, and proteins, is essential. The integrity of the hair strands may be preserved by employing good hair care techniques, including careful handling, the use of appropriate hair products, and avoiding excessive heat or chemical treatments.

A healthy lifestyle in general might benefit hair health. A healthy body may assist in healthy hair development. This is made possible by regular exercise, stress management, and enough sleep. It's crucial to keep in mind that each individual has different hair, so what works for one person may not necessarily work for another. It's important to find a hair care regimen and products that work for your particular hair type and requirements.

On the other hand, hair loss may be upsetting and may be caused by a number of different factors. Genes, hormone imbalances, illnesses, drugs, and lifestyle choices may all have an impact on it. The best treatment choices must be made after establishing the cause of hair loss. A dermatologist or other healthcare expert may provide insightful advice and assist in developing a tailored strategy to manage hair loss problems.

We shall go more deeply into the worlds of healthy hair and hair loss in this tutorial.

We'll look at the elements that contribute to having healthy hair, talk about the most frequent reasons why people lose their hair, and provide some tips for managing and preventing hair loss. We may take proactive measures to preserve healthy, resilient hair throughout our lifetimes by better understanding the complex systems behind hair health.Based on their texture, thickness, and curl pattern, the various hair types may be distinguished from one another.

THE FOLLOWING LIST OF TYPICAL HAIR TYPES INCLUDES METHODS FOR IDENTIFYING EACH ONE

First, straight hairTexture: Straight hair has little to no curl or wave and is typically smooth.It may range from being fine to being coarse in thickness.Straight hair has a propensity to be lustrous, light-reflective, and less frizzy.

2. Wavy hair: texture: wavy hair has loose curls or a small "S" form.Thickness: There are many thicknesses available.Wavy hair may be dryer or more volumized, and it is also more prone to frizz. From mild to more obvious, the wave's strength might change.

3. Curly hair may produce tight or loose curls, spirals, or coils, depending on the texture.Thickness: There are many thicknesses available.Curly hair is more prone to tangling, frizz, and dryness than straight hair. For it to stay defined and in form, it could need extra moisture and certain styling methods.

4. Coily or Kinky HairCoily or kinky hair has curly strands that are firmly coiled or curled in zigzag patterns.It may be anything from fine to coarse in thickness.Curly or kinky hair is prone to dryness, is often packed tightly, and may shorten as it becomes dry. Regular hydration, safeguarding, and delicate handling are necessary.

You should be aware that different people have different kinds of hair. An individual could, for instance, have straight hair at the roots that progressively turns wavy or curly towards the ends. Having a mix of several hair kinds on various parts of the head is also a possibility.

CAUSES OF HAIR LOSS

Alopecia, another name for hair loss, may afflict people of all ages. Numerous variables, including genetics, hormone changes, illnesses, a person's lifestyle, and environmental factors, might contribute to hair loss. The following are some typical reasons for hair loss in both young and elderly people:

Genetic Factors: Hereditary pattern baldness, also known as androgenetic alopecia, is the most frequent cause of hair loss in both men and women. This disorder, which is influenced by a mix of hormonal and genetic factors, may cause gradual hair loss over time.

Hormonal Changes: Unbalanced hormone levels may be a factor in hair loss. Male pattern baldness in males may be brought on by an increase in the hormone dihydrotestosterone (DHT), which is generated from testosterone. Hair thinning or shedding in women may be brought on by hormonal changes brought on by illnesses including polycystic ovarian syndrome (PCOS), pregnancy, childbirth, menopause, or other factors.

Medical Conditions: Several ailments, including the following, may cause hair loss:Alopecia areata is an autoimmune disorder that causes patchy hair loss as a consequence of the immune system erroneously attacking hair follicles.Disorders of the thyroid: An overactive or underactive thyroid gland may interfere with the cycle of hair development and result in hair loss.Scalp infections: Hair loss may result from bacterial or fungal infections of the scalp.Trichotillomania is a psychiatric condition that causes obsessive hair pulling, which results in observable hair loss.

Drugs and medical procedures: A number of drugs and medical procedures may result in either temporary or permanent hair loss. These include several pharmaceuticals used to treat autoimmune diseases, hormone treatments, radiation therapy, and chemotherapy agents.

Nutritional Deficiencies: Hair health may be impacted, and hair loss can result from inadequate consumption of vital minerals such as iron, zinc, biotin, and vitamins A, D, and E.

Stress and Trauma: Telogen effluvium, a kind of hair loss, may be brought on by physical or mental stress, trauma, or important life events. Premature hair follicle resting phases brought on by this disorder result in severe hair loss and thinning.

Hairstyling and Hair Practices: Hair breakage and traction alopecia, which results in hair loss, can be brought on by certain hairstyling practices, such as the frequent use of heat styling tools, tight hairstyles (such as ponytails or braids), chemical treatments (like perming or relaxing), and aggressive brushing or combing.

Age-related factors: As people age, their rate of hair development may slow down and their hair follicles may become weaker and less active. Hair loss or thinning may be caused by this normal aging process.

Autoimmune Conditions: Some autoimmune conditions, such lupus or alopecia universalis, may result in hair loss by damaging hair follicles or interfering with the hair development cycle.

Traumatic Hair Loss: Physical harm to the scalp, such as burns, wounds, or surgical operations, may cause hair loss in the afflicted regions.

Environmental variables: Exposure to environmental variables, such as toxins, pollutants, and harsh chemicals, may weaken the hair shaft and cause hair loss or damage.

Poor Hair Care Practices: incorrect hair care, such as excessive use of harsh hair products, frequent bleaching or dyeing, and incorrect handling or style methods, may cause hair loss or breaking.

Significant and Rapid Weight Loss: Hair loss may result from nutritional inadequacies and hormonal imbalances, which are typically linked to crash diets or eating disorders.

Medications and Medical Treatments: As a side effect, several medications, including blood thinners, antidepressants, and antifungal agents, may result in hair loss. Radiation therapy and other medical procedures may also cause temporary or permanent hair loss in certain places.

Prolonged or severe sickness, major operations, or substantial physical stress may all lead to hair loss. Telogen effluvium is the term used to describe this kind of hair loss, which often occurs temporarily.

Hormonal Imbalances: Changes in hormone levels may be a factor in hair loss. Hair thinning or shedding is a symptom of a number of illnesses, including polycystic ovarian syndrome (PCOS), thyroid abnormalities (hyper- or hypothyroidism), and menopausal hormone changes.

Scalp disorders: Some disorders of the scalp, such as scalp psoriasis, seborrheic dermatitis, or fungal infections (such as ringworm), may inflame the hair follicles and harm them, which can lead to hair loss.

Emotional and psychological Contributing issues: Psychological issues, including stress, worry, or emotional anguish, may cause hair loss. Significant hair loss may result from illnesses like trichotillomania (a disease characterized by obsessive hair pulling), excessive hair twisting, and neurotic behaviors.

Chemotherapy and radiation: Since they target rapidly dividing cells, including hair follicles, cancer therapies like chemotherapy and radiation therapy may result in hair loss. Hair often grows back after cancer treatment; thus, hair loss is typically just temporary.

Smoking may damage hair health and be a factor in hair loss, according to research. Smoking lowers the blood supply to the hair follicles, which may cause them to become frail and cause hair thinning.
Poor blood circulation: hair follicle activity may be affected, and hair loss can be exacerbated by inadequate blood flow to the

scalp. The blood flow to the scalp might be impacted by factors including a sedentary lifestyle, tightly styled hair, or underlying vascular disorders.

Hair Pulling and Traction: Traction alopecia is the medical term for hair loss and damage caused by habitual hair pulling, such as in trichotillomania instances, or persistent strain on the hair from tight hairstyles like braids, weaves, or extensions.

Remember that the underlying cause must be addressed before treating or managing hair loss. A dermatologist or healthcare provider should be consulted if you have noticeable or worrying hair loss in order to get an accurate diagnosis and create a treatment plan that is specifically tailored to your needs.

Nutritional deficiencies may affect hair health and cause hair loss. This is due to inadequate consumption or absorption of vital nutrients. The development and quality of hair may be impacted by nutritional deficiencies in a number of nutrients, including biotin, vitamin D, zinc, and iron.

Excessive Styling or Chemical Treatments: The use of blow dryers, flat irons, or curling irons too often or vigorously may weaken and damage hair due to heat. Similarly, regular hair dyeing, relaxing, or other chemical treatments may cause hair loss and breakage if used excessively.

Drug Side Effects: Hair loss may occur as a side effect of various drugs, including some beta-blockers, antidepressants, and anticoagulants. Consult your healthcare practitioner for other alternatives if you think your medicine is making you bald.

Radiation Exposure: High doses of radiation, like those given during cancer radiation treatment or from radiation spills, may harm hair follicles and cause hair loss in the affected regions.

Anemia: Hair loss may be a symptom of anemia, which is defined by a lack of hemoglobin or red blood cells. Hair loss and thinning are known to be exacerbated by anemia caused by iron deficiency, in particular.

Autoimmune Disorders: A number of autoimmune disorders, including systemic lupus erythematosus (SLE) and autoimmune thyroiditis, may result in hair loss because the immune system incorrectly attacks the hair follicles.

Environmental Toxins: Exposure to certain environmental toxins, such as heavy metals, pollution, or chemicals, may harm hair follicles and cause hair loss.

Trichotillomania: Trichotillomania is a psychiatric illness that is defined by a compulsive impulse to pluck out one's hair, leaving behind considerable hair loss.

CHAPTER 2

PROMOTING HAIR GROWTH INVOLVES

maintaining a healthy scalp and providing proper care for your hair.

Balanced Diet: Ensure your diet includes a variety of nutrients that promote hair health, such as protein, biotin, vitamins A, C, and E, zinc, and omega-3 fatty acids. Include foods like eggs, fish, nuts, fruits, vegetables, and whole grains.

Scalp Massage: Regularly massaging your scalp can help improve blood circulation, which in turn promotes hair growth. Use your fingertips to massage your scalp in circular motions for a few minutes daily.

Gentle Hair Care: Avoid harsh treatments, excessive heat styling, and tight hairstyles that can damage your hair. Use a wide-toothed comb or a brush with soft bristles to prevent hair breakage.

Regular Trimming: Although it may sound counterintuitive, getting regular trims (every 6–8 weeks) helps prevent split ends and breakage, allowing your hair to grow healthier.

Avoid overwashing: washing your hair too frequently can strip it of natural oils, which are essential for healthy hair growth. Aim to wash your hair every 2-3 days, or as needed, using a gentle shampoo and conditioner.

Deep Conditioning: Apply a deep conditioner or hair mask once a week to nourish and moisturize your hair. Look for products that contain ingredients like argan oil, coconut oil, or shea butter.

Avoid Excessive Heat: Minimize the use of heat-styling tools such as straighteners, curling irons, and blow dryers. Excessive heat can damage the hair shaft and impede hair growth. If you must use heat, apply a heat-protectant spray and use the lowest setting.

Protect from Sun and Pollution: Shield your hair from excessive sun exposure and pollution, as they can weaken the hair and hinder growth. Wear a hat or use a scarf to protect your hair when outdoors.

Stay Hydrated: Drink an adequate amount of water daily to keep your body and hair hydrated. Hydration is important for overall hair health.

Manage stress: Chronic stress can negatively impact hair growth. Practice stress management techniques such as exercise, meditation, deep breathing, or engaging in hobbies to promote overall well-being.

Consult a Dermatologist: If you're experiencing significant hair loss or have concerns about your scalp's health, it's best to consult a dermatologist or a trichologist for a professional evaluation and personalized advice.

Use Hair Growth Products: Seek out hair growth products that include minoxidil, an FDA-approved chemical that encourages hair renewal. It's crucial to use these products regularly and according to the directions if you want to see results in terms of promoting hair growth.

Consider using essential oils: Some essential oils have been linked to the stimulation of hair growth. For instance, lavender oil, peppermint oil, and rosemary oil might all help increase blood flow and encourage hair growth. Massage your scalp with a few drops of diluted essential oil mixed with a carrier oil, such as coconut oil or jojoba oil.

Take supplements: Particularly if you have dietary deficits, several supplements might promote hair growth. To find out whether and how much vitamins like biotin, vitamin D, or iron are right for you, speak with a medical expert.

Quit Smoking: Smoking inhibits the development of hair by tightening blood vessels and decreasing circulation. Better hair health might result from quitting smoking or avoiding secondhand smoke.

Protect your hair at night: Before bed, wrap your hair in a silk or satin scarf or use a satin or silk pillowcase. In comparison to cotton, these fabrics provide less friction, which might lessen the likelihood of hair breakage and damage.

Take into account low-level laser treatment: Red light therapy, commonly referred to as low-level laser therapy, has shown potential for accelerating hair growth. In order to activate the hair follicles, devices that transmit red light onto the scalp are used. To learn more about this possibility, speak with a dermatologist or other member of the medical community.

Refrain from Excessive Hair Manipulation: Constant pulling and tugging on your hair may damage and break it. Avoid tight hairstyles that cause strain on the hair and use gentle techniques when combing or styling your hair.

Exercise regularly: This may increase circulation throughout the body, especially to the scalp, which may help with hair development. Exercise and other activities that increase heart rate and blood flow should be done.

Be Patient and Consistent: Keep in mind that hair development takes time, so don't expect results right away. It's crucial to maintain consistency in your hair care practice and allow results to develop.

NATURAL WAY TO BOOST HAIR GROWTH

When applied directly to the hair and scalp, a number of natural substances have been shown to promote hair growth. Below are a few possibilities:

1. Aloe vera is a hydrating plant that also possesses enzymes that encourage hair development. Apply aloe vera leaf gel straight to the scalp after extracting the gel. Before washing it off, let it sit for about 30 minutes.

2. Coconut oil: Coconut oil is well-known for its hydrating and nourishing qualities. Your scalp and hair should be well coated in

heated coconut oil as you massage it in. Overnight, leave it on, and the next morning, wash it off.

3. Onion juice: Because onion juice is high in sulfur, it might increase blood flow to hair follicles and encourage hair growth. Get the juice from an onion by blending it. Before fully washing, apply the juice to your scalp and let it sit for 30 minutes.

4. Rosemary oil: Rosemary oil is claimed to energize hair follicles and encourage hair growth. Several drops of rosemary oil should be combined with a carrier oil, such as coconut or olive oil. Then, wash it off with water after at least 30 minutes of massaging the mixture into your scalp.

5. Green tea: The antioxidants in green tea may aid in promoting hair development. Strong green tea should be brewed and allowed to cool. It should be applied to your scalp, let sit for an hour, and then rinsed out. Just keep in mind that although using these natural compounds may help increase hair growth, specific outcomes may vary. To promote general hair health, it's also important to maintain a healthy lifestyle, consume a balanced diet, and take care of your hair. Consult with a dermatologist or other healthcare provider for individualized guidance if you have any scalp disorders that need to be treated or worry about hair loss.

6. Castor oil: Castor oil is a great source of vitamin E, minerals, and fatty acids that feed hair follicles and encourage hair development. Castor oil may be applied to the scalp by massaging heated oil into it. The following morning, wash it off.

7. Peppermint oil: This oil has a cooling effect and may assist in increasing blood flow to the scalp, which encourages hair growth. Apply a few drops of peppermint oil to your scalp after blending it with a carrier oil. Before washing it off, let it sit for 20 to 30 minutes.

8. Fenugreek seeds: Fenugreek seeds are high in proteins and nicotinic acid, which may help strengthen hair follicles and encourage hair growth. Fenugreek seeds

should be soaked overnight and then ground into a paste the following morning. Apply the paste to your scalp and let it sit for 30 minutes before giving it a good rinse.

9. Apple cider vinegar: By balancing the pH of the scalp, apple cider vinegar may encourage thicker, healthier hair growth. After washing your hair, make an equal mixture of apple cider vinegar and water and use it as a final rinse. Before washing it off, let it sit for a while.

10. Henna: Henna is a natural hair conditioner that helps strengthen hair and encourage growth. Make a paste out of henna powder and water, then let it sit for a few hours. Apply the paste to your hair, then

let it sit in place for a few hours before washing it off.

11. Lemon juice: Lemon juice is high in vitamin C, which may encourage hair growth. Apply freshly squeezed lemon juice and water to your scalp.

12. Hibiscus: Hibiscus blossoms are said to strengthen hair and encourage hair development.

13. Egg mask: Eggs are a great source of biotin and protein, both of which are necessary for healthy hair development.

14. Jojoba oil: Jojoba oil closely mirrors the natural oils generated by the scalp, making

it a wonderful alternative for hydrating and encouraging hair development.

15. Fenugreek oil: Made from fenugreek seeds, fenugreek oil helps strengthen hair follicles and encourage hair growth.

CHAPTER 3

HOW TO APPLY

1. Aloe vera: Apply the gel from an aloe vera leaf immediately to the scalp. Before washing it off with water, you may keep it on for around 30 minutes.

2. Warm coconut oil and massage it into your scalp and hair. For deep conditioning, leave it on all night. The next morning, wash it off with a gentle shampoo.

3. To extract onion juice, blend an onion. Directly apply the juice to your scalp and give it a little massage. Before fully washing with a gentle shampoo, let it sit for 30 minutes.

4. Rosemary oil: Combine a few drops of rosemary oil with a carrier oil, such as coconut oil or olive oil. Use circular movements to massage the mixture into your scalp. Before rinsing it off with a gentle shampoo, let it sit for at least 30 minutes.

5. Green tea: Prepare a pot of strong green tea and let it cool. Apply the cooled green tea to your scalp and hair, being careful to get the roots wet. Before washing it off with water, let it sit for an hour.

6. Castor oil: Apply warmed castor oil to your scalp. For a few minutes, gently massage it in to encourage absorption. Leave it on all night, then remove it in the morning with a gentle shower.

7. Peppermint oil: Combine a few drops of peppermint oil with a carrier oil, such as coconut oil or olive oil. Massage the mixture into your scalp. Before washing it off with a gentle shampoo, let it sit for 20 to 30 minutes.

8. Soak fenugreek seeds overnight. Make a paste out of them the following morning, then rub it on your scalp. Before properly washing with water, leave it on for 30 minutes.

9. Apple cider vinegar: Combine equal amounts of apple cider vinegar and water. Use the combination as a last rinse after washing your hair, making sure to cover

both your scalp and hair. Before washing it off with water, let it sit for a few minutes.

10.   Henna: Prepare a thick paste by combining henna powder and water. Starting at the roots and moving to the ends, apply the paste to your hair. Rinse it off with water after leaving it on for a few hours or until it has fully dried.

11. Lemon juice: Use a cotton ball or spray bottle to apply freshly squeezed lemon juice to your scalp. Before washing it off with water, let it sit for 15 to 20 minutes.

12. Hibiscus: To make a paste, crush some hibiscus flowers and combine them with coconut oil or olive oil. Apply the paste to your scalp and hair, then let it sit for an

hour before washing it off with a gentle shampoo.

13. Use an egg as a hair and scalp mask by whisking the egg well. Leave it on for 30 to 60 minutes, then rinse it off with cold water and a light shampoo.

14. Jojoba oil: Apply jojoba oil evenly throughout your hair and scalp by massaging it thoroughly. For deep conditioning, let it on for a few hours or over the night. Then, remove it with a light shampoo.

15. Fenugreek oil: Massage fenugreek oil into your scalp and hair, then keep it on for several hours or overnight. Use water and a gentle wash to remove it.

CONCLUSION

The length of time it takes to see effects may vary based on a number of variables, including your own hair growth rate, the general health of your hair, how consistently you use the product, and the particular state of your hair and scalp. Some individuals could show changes in only a few weeks, while others might need many months of consistent usage to see effects. In general, while employing natural therapies for hair growth, it's necessary to have reasonable expectations and be patient. The benefits of these chemicals take time to become apparent since hair development is a gradual process. Additionally, keep in mind that these natural solutions function best when used as a component of an all-encompassing hair care regimen that also includes a balanced diet, enough hydration, and effective hair care techniques. When employing natural medicines, consistency is essential. To give them a chance to function well, it is advised to use them often, preferably a few times each week or as indicated. To monitor any alterations or advancements over time, you can also think about maintaining a hair growth log. It's recommended to speak with a dermatologist or other healthcare provider if you have any underlying scalp issues or worries about hair loss. Based on your unique requirements, they may provide an accurate diagnosis and suggest suitable therapies or further interventions. In the end, practice patience and consistency, and provide your hair and scalp with the necessary care.